TLC DIET
7 DAY MEAL PLAN FOR RAPID WEIGHT LOSS

BY TIMOTHY PYKE

Copyright © 2015 RIGS Publishing

To subscribe to Tim's latest work and get some FREE eBooks go to:

TimothyPyke.com

ABOUT THIS BOOK

The National Institute of Health created the Therapeutic Lifestyle Changes (TLC) diet as a plan to lower the levels of low-density lipoprotein (LDL) cholesterol. The TLC diet is endorsed by the American Heart Association as an effective method of decreasing the risk of heart disease.

The TLC diet is not just focused on weight-loss; it also focuses on building a healthy lifestyle and sustaining an ideal body weight. If you are looking for an easy to follow and straightforward diet or you want to live a happy and healthy lifestyle, then this is the diet for you.

TABLE OF CONTENTS

CHAPTER 1: INTRODUCTION TO NUTRITION

The National Cholesterol Education Program formed the TLC Diet in 2001 with the intent to educate individuals about fat, cholesterol and heart disease. The TLC diet aims to lower the quantity of saturated fats in your diet, which in turn decreases your LDL cholesterol – the 'bad' cholesterol.

FATS & CHOLESTEROL

LDL cholesterol contributes to plaque - a concentrated, rigid deposit that can clog arteries and reduce their flexibility. This condition is known as atherosclerosis. Excess plaque can lead to the formation of an arterial clot – sometimes resulting in a heart attack or stroke. Peripheral Artery Disease can develop when a build-up of plaque narrows some of the arteries delivering blood to the legs.

Research has shown that high-density lipoprotein (HDL) – the 'good' cholesterol – carries LDL cholesterol away from the arteries and back to the liver where it is degraded and expelled from the body. Exchanging saturated fats for mono- or poly-unsaturated fats leads to a reduction in LDL and an increase in HDL cholesterol. The ratio of HDL to LDL is an indicator of overall arterial health and doctors often measure this ratio in screening for disease. A healthy ratio of HDL to LDL cholesterol protects against heart attack and stroke.

Trans-fats are created by an artificial process that adds hydrogen to liquid vegetable oils to make them more solid. The primary source of trans-fats in processed food is "partially hydrogenated oils" - look for them in the ingredients list on the back of food packaging. Trans-fats raise your LDL cholesterol levels and lower your good HDL cholesterol levels, increasing your risk of heart disease and stroke. Trans-fats are also linked to a higher risk of developing type-2 diabetes. In November 2013, the U.S. Food and Drug

Administration (FDA) stated that partially hydrogenated oils are no longer Generally Recognized as Safe in human food.

One key imperative of the TLC diet is avoiding trans-fats. Trans-fats can be found in many foods – including doughnuts, cakes, pie crusts, frozen pizzas, cookies, crackers, biscuits, stick margarines and other spreads.

Saturated fats are simply fat molecules that have no double bonds between carbon molecules resulting in a lengthier, stiffer structure. Saturated fats are typically solid at room temperature. Ingesting saturated fats increases your LDL or bad cholesterol and reduces your HDL or good cholesterol. Saturated fats occur naturally in many foods. The majority come mainly from animal sources, including meat and dairy products such as fatty beef, chicken skin, cream, and butter. Baked goods and fried foods can also contain high levels of saturated fats. Some plant oils, such as palm oil, palm kernel oil and coconut oil, also contain saturated fats.

You should replace saturated fats with foods high in monounsaturated or polyunsaturated fats. This means eating foods made with liquid vegetable oils, and eating fish and nuts. You should replace some of the meat you eat with beans or legumes.

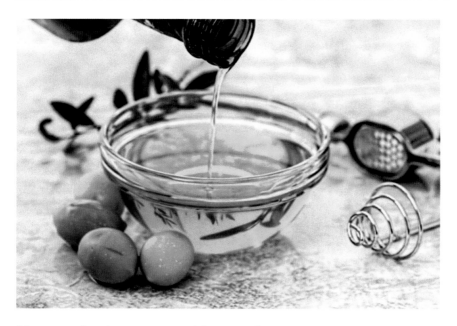

Mono- and poly-unsaturated fats are fat molecules that have one or more double bonds between carbon molecules. This results in a kinked and loser structure than that of saturated fats. Oils that contain mono- and poly-unsaturated fats are usually liquid at room temperature but solidify when cooled. Olive oil contains both mono- and poly-unsaturated fats.

Unsaturated fats reduce bad cholesterol levels which can lower your risk of heart disease and stroke. They also provide nutrients to help develop and maintain your body's cells. Eating food made with oils rich in unsaturated fats will also add vitamin E to the diet - an antioxidant which helps battle many diseases related to cellular oxidative stress.

Omega-3 and omega-6 fatty acids need special mention here as they can only be obtained through food yet are essential to the proper bodily function. These polyunsaturated fats help both the brain and heart. Sources of Omega-3 fatty acid are fatty fish, canola oil, walnuts, olives and flax seeds. The type obtained from fatty fish is superior to that from nuts and fruits. Other sources include parsley, Brussels sprouts, spinach and kale among vegetables.

Among non-vegetable sources, we have salmon, sardines, oysters, herring, lake trout and fish oil.

SUGARS & CARBOHYDRATES

Sugars, starches and fiber are the three types of carbohydrates in your food. Carbohydrates are classed as either simple or complex based on their chemical structure and rate of digestion and absorption into the body. Eating foods with high simple carbohydrate content may lead to an increase in your LDL levels. Simple carbohydrates (or simple sugars) are digested more rapidly than complex carbohydrates and cause a blood glucose spike shortly after being eaten. Refined sugars and added sugars are examples of simple sugars. Added sugars increase your caloric intake but don't provide many other nutrients – they are empty calories. However, simple sugars are also found in fruits and milk which provide valuable nutrients, minerals and fiber as well.

Complex carbohydrates are digested slowly and will not spike your blood stream with glucose. This results in a steady supply of energy to your muscles, liver, brain and other organs. Refined grains - such as white flour or white rice - contain complex carbohydrates. However, due to their processing they lack many nutrients and fiber. Instead, opt for unrefined whole grains – these will contain the vital nutrients and fiber. Fiber helps your digestive system work properly. While the fiber itself cannot be digested by humans it does help you feel fuller for longer.

During digestion, carbohydrates are broken down to simple sugars and absorbed into the bloodstream. The pancreas detects the rise in blood sugar levels and secretes the hormone insulin. Insulin triggers cells to take in sugar from the blood where it is used as an energy source, stored as glycogen or converted into fats. Diabetes is a disease where the body has difficulty regulating its insulin levels.

Overall, try to limit foods that have high processed or refined simple sugar content - these foods provide extra calories (which may lead to weight gain) but they have no nutritional value. Focus on getting complex carbohydrates and healthy nutrients in your diet by eating more fruits and vegetables, beans, lentils and dried peas, whole-grain rice, breads and cereals.

Chapter 2: Adopting the TLC Diet for Better Health

The Role of Fats in our Metabolism

The truth about fat is rather astonishing because our body needs fat to survive. Fat functions as protection for the internal organs from physical injury; it insulates the body minimizing heat loss. Fats help dissolve vitamins A, K, E and D and for storage in the liver and adipose (fatty) tissue until required. Vitamins C and B complex are water soluble. Yet, to transport the other four vitamins, we need fats. The point is that we choose good fats to do the work!

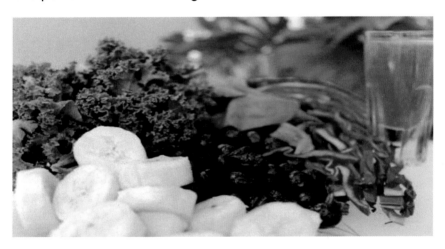

We need these vitamins in small amounts only. In the TLC Diet, we choose foods that provide the requisite amounts of these vitamins and fats. Do you know just what these vitamins do? Vitamin K helps in blood clotting and formation of bones and tissues. Vitamin E is by contrast an agent that prevents clotting as it is an antioxidant. Vitamin D along with Vitamin C helps the body develop healthy bones. Vitamin A helps develop keen eyesight and helps the reproductive and immune system. It helps tooth and bone development and assists in the functioning of the lungs, heart and kidneys.

Nutrient	Used For	Present In
Vitamin A	Eye, immune system, development of cells, healthy skin	Vegetables that are dark green in color; orange vegetables such as carrots, sweet potatoes, kale, cantaloupe, papayas
Vitamin D	Bone building and strength	Sunshine, egg yolk, soy milk, orange juice
Vitamin B12	Red blood cells, nerve cell function, guard against anemia	Egg, red meat, fish, cheese, poultry, cereal, liver
Thiamin	Necessary ingredient for functioning of nervous system, heart, muscles – helps convert carbohydrates to energy	Lean meat, pasta, bread, peas, soy, whole grains
Riboflavin	Red blood cell production, converts carbohydrates to energy, general growth	Egg, legumes, meat, leafy green vegetables like broccoli, nuts and dairy products
Vitamin C	Collagen that keeps the body cells together needs this vitamin, also by teeth, bones and blood vessels	Citrus fruits, spinach, broccoli, guava, strawberries tomatoes and peppers
Vitamin E	Antioxidant that prevents damage to cells	Vegetable oils, avocados, green leafy

		vegetables, whole grains, nuts and wheat germ
Vitamin B6	Assists in brain and nerve function, digestion of proteins, manufacture of RBC, stabilize blood sugar, make antibodies	Banana, potato, fish, egg, fortified cereal, spinach, red meat, chick peas and nuts
Niacin	Converts food to energy, helps keep the skin healthy, assist nerve function	Poultry, fish, meat, peanuts and cereal
Folate	Makes RBCs, helps make DNA	Liver, orange juice, asparagus, legumes, green leafy vegetables
Calcium	Blood clotting, bone health, muscle contraction	Milk, cheese, yogurt, kale and fortified cereals
Chromium	Control blood sugar levels	Poultry, fish, potato, broccoli
Fiber	Lowers LDL, gives satiation, stimulates bowel movement, maintain blood sugar level	Peas, beans, fruits, oatmeal
Copper	Helps in processing iron	Lentils, peas, beans, vegetables and fruits
Fluoride	Helps in digestion, maintains blood sugar levels, makes you feel	Fluoridated water, seafood

	full	
Iodine	Helps thyroid hormone production	Turkey, beans, soy beans, lentils, spinach
Folate	Keeps heart healthy, cell development, prevents birth defects	Dark green leafy vegetables, whole grain cereals
Manganese	Enzyme production, bone formation	Tea, legumes, whole grains, nuts
Potassium	Reduces kidney stones, control blood pressure	Soybeans, yogurt, milk, bananas, potatoes
Selenium	Needed for thyroid hormone, prevents cell damage	Seafood, Brazil nuts, dairy food, organ meat
Sodium	Fluid balance	Table salt

FINDING YOUR ENERGY REQUIREMENTS

Our body requires energy to carry out basic metabolic activities. This includes breathing, blood circulation, maintaining the central nervous system, digestion and tissue repair. This amount of energy (when you are doing nothing) goes by the name of Basal Metabolic Rate (BMR). We get energy from food we eat. Eating right thus helps our metabolism get the most energy and function in the best manner.

The BMR depends on factors like age, height and weight of the person. Here you have the revised Harris-Benedict equation:

For men: $P = (13.397m + 4.799h - 5.677a + 88.362)$ Cal/day

For women: $P = (9.247m + 3.098h - 4.330a + 44.7593)$ Cal/day

Legend: m - weight in Kg, h - height in cm, a - age in years

You can arrive at your BMR value by using your own values in the formula. For example, a lady 76 years old, weighing 53 kg and 156 cm tall would have a BMR of 689.06 Cal/day. A male who is 52 years old, weighing 71 kg and 165 cm tall would have a BMR of 1530 Cal/day. So if you were a male on a 2,500 Cal/day diet, you would have surplus of 970 Cal that would be used to walk around and do work.

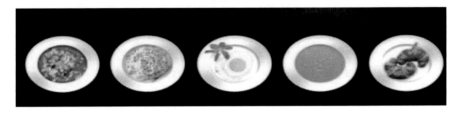

When you do more activity, you use more than 2,500 Cal (include your BMR). Then the body converts stored fat to energy resulting in weight loss.

Activity	Energy Utilized (Cal/kg/hour)
Sleeping	0.9
Walking (5km/h)	2.9
Light Moderate Home Exercises	3.5
Sexual Activity	5.8
Jogging	7
Running in place	8
Rope Jumping	10

If you weigh 70 kg, multiply the above factor by 70. Say, you walk for ½ hour, have sex for 20 minutes and go jogging for 40 minutes, you would need:

(0.5 * 2.9 * 70) + (1/3 * 5.8 * 70) + (2/3 * 7 * 70) = 564 Cal

If you had 1000 Cal excess, you have now used up 564 Cal. The body stores the excess energy (346 Cal) as fats in the liver and fatty tissue. Or you can take a longer walk for 90 minutes more and use up all the energy. Remember, approximations form the base for the calculations. If you feel hungry at the end of the day then stick with the diet for one more day. You should feel better and healthier. If not you can adjust the amount of food a little every day. You reach the level where you have complete satisfaction.

CHAPTER 3: TLC DIET GUIDELINES

Nutrient	Recommended Intake
Saturated fat	<19 g
Polyunsaturated fat	28 g
Monounsaturated fat	56 g
Carbohydrates	165 g
Fiber	25 g
Potassium	4.7 g
Salt	<1.5 g
Protein	23 g
Vitamin B12	2.4 micrograms
Vitamin D	15 micrograms
Cholesterol	0.2 g
Total Calories	2,500 Cal

Calcium

This is vital to form and preserve the bones. Besides, it makes muscles and blood vessels function in correct manner. Many people in the United States unfortunately get insufficient amount through their diet. The recommendation for females over the age of 50 is to have around 1,150 milligrams of calcium per day.

Fiber

This diet ensures you get adequate amounts of dietary fiber. It promotes nutrient absorption in the intestines, and helps you feel fuller for longer. Fruits, vegetables, beans and whole grains are major sources of fiber.

Potassium

An acceptable potassium amount in the diet counters the power of salt. Salt elevates blood pressure. It also discontinues bone loss and reduces the risk of developing stones in the kidney. It is difficult getting the suggested daily 4,700 milligrams from this nourishment alone.

Sodium

TLC keeps tight rein on the intake of sodium which should be at most 2,300 milligrams per day. A 1,500 milligram limit is set for African-American people aged 51 years and above. The same goes for people with hypertension, diabetes, and chronic kidney diseases.

Vitamin B-12

Adults must aim for 2. 4 micrograms as it is the critical limit for proper cell metabolism. Yogurt is a source of this vitamin.

Vitamin D

Adults getting insufficient sunlight need 15 micrograms as a nutrition supplement. This lessens the risk of bone fractures.

The TLC Diet is a three-layered regimen consisting of food, exercise and medicine. Taking multivitamins if necessary may also be beneficial – consult your physician to find the right supplement for you.

CHAPTER 4: TLC MISTAKES

Always inspect the nutritional information of the food you eat for cholesterol and fat content. Stay away from those that have trans-fat or partly hydrogenated vegetable oils. You find them in compact margarine, vegetable shortening, chips, biscuits, and cookies. Control the use of dietary oils and saturated fat. Examples are palm and coconut oils, bacon drippings, and butter.

Instead, you can opt for soft margarine or vegetable oils. Restrict fatty animal meats by avoiding food such as bologna, hot dogs, steaks, pastrami, corned pork and beef, and other processed foods. Replace these foods with skinned turkey or chicken and fish. Experiment with quite a few meat-free recipes of peas, beans, pasta and rice. Just remember to limit fish, meat and poultry to at most two portions - around 140 grams - daily.

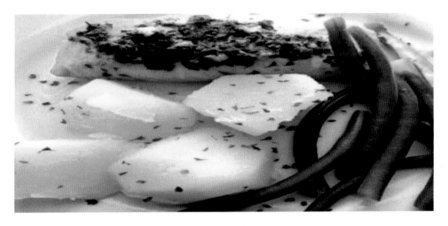

Also, avoid dairy products with more than one percent fat, like creams, cheeses, cakes. The same applies to creamy toppings made from palm or coconut oils. Instead, set your sights on low-fat or fat-free milk and cheeses. Be wary of breads, snack wafers, muffins, croissants, and cakes - these are often baked with trans-fat or regular milk. Check out low-fat baked foods and enjoy it with vegetable garnishing, sauce or light toppings.

When you eat out avoid burgers, chips, wedges, tacos or anything deep-fried. They are high in total fat. Instead, select roasted chicken without skin in sandwiches, and salads having low-fat vinaigrette. Ask the waiter to exclude the high-fat salad dressings and cheese from your salad.

When cooking, avoid using butter and high-fat sauces. Bake, microwave, steam, poach or sauté your dishes and use vegetable oils high in mono- and poly-unsaturated fats such as olive oil, safflower oil and canola oil. Use non-stick pans instead of extra oil.

Refrigerate casseroles and broths overnight – the fat will float to the top of the gravy and solidify. Strain out this fat before reheating. Cut salt from soups, grilled chicken, vegetables and seafood – or replace with low-sodium salts or herbs and spices to add flavor. You can also use bits of smoked turkey meat to add a savory punch while keeping fat content low. Skinless chicken thighs are a good substitute for chicken neck.

CHAPTER 5: MEAL PLAN WITH RECIPES

DAY 1

Breakfast

1 cup Raisin oatmeal

1 medium English muffin using 2 teaspoons soft margarine and a tablespoon of jelly

1 cup Honeydew melon

1 cup Calcium fortified orange juice

1 cup Coffee with 2 tablespoons non-fat milk

Raising Oatmeal

Preparation time: 3 minutes

Cooking time: 2 minutes

Ingredients:

1 cup non-fat milk

1 serving old-fashioned rolled oats

¼ cup raisins

Directions:

Boil the rolled oats, add the milk, and top with the raisins.

Lunch

1 Roast beef sandwich

1 cup Pasta salad using ¾ cup of pasta noodles, 1/4 cup mixed veggies, and 2 teaspoons of olive oil

1 medium Apple

1 cup unsweetened iced tea

Roast Beef Sandwich

Preparation time: 2 minutes

Cooking time: 5 minutes

Ingredients:

1 medium whole wheat bun

2 ounces lean beef

1 ounce sliced low-fat Swiss cheese

2 leaves Romaine lettuce

2 medium slices of tomato

2 teaspoons mustard

Directions:

First you must heat nonstick skillet above medium temperature. Grill the lean beef until golden brown. Flip and top it with cheese until it starts to melt. Cut the bun in half and on each side, spread the mustard and top each with lettuce and tomato. Place the cooked beef with cheese in the middle and enjoy the sandwich.

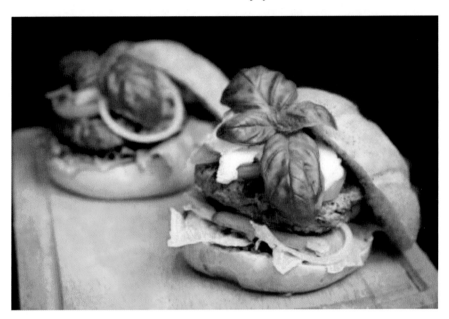

Dinner

Orange Rice Topping

½ cup Corn kernels with a teaspoon of soft margarine

½ cup Broccoli with a teaspoon of soft margarine

1 small Bread roll with a teaspoon of soft margarine

1 cup Strawberries topped with ½ cup low-fat frozen yogurt

1 cup non-fat milk

Orange Rice Topping

Preparation time: 7 minutes

Cooking time: 20 minutes

Ingredients:

3 ounces peeled and sliced seedless oranges

2 teaspoon olive oil

1 tablespoon Parmesan cheese

2 cups water

1½ cups Rice

Directions:

Wash the rice and cook inside a rice cooker using 2 cups of water. In a nonstick pan, heat over medium fire the olive oil. Add orange slices and cheese and sauté for a minute or two before putting it on top of fresh boiled rice.

Snack

2 cups of Popcorn cooked with a tablespoon of canola oil, 1 cup canned Peaches and 1 cup Water

Day 1 breakdown

Nutrition Facts	
	Amount
Calories	2543 g
Proteins	105 g
Fats	78 g
Saturated fats	19 g
Monounsaturated fats	39 g
Polyunsaturated fats	20 g
Cholesterol	139 mg
Carbohydrates	351 g
Fiber	32 g
Sodium	1800 mg

DAY 2

Breakfast

Preparation time: 2 minutes

Cooking time: 3 minutes

1 cup Strawberry oatmeal using a cup of non-fat milk and ¼ cup sliced fresh strawberries

1 cup Melon cubes

1 cup calcium fortified Pineapple juice

1 cup Tea with 2 tablespoons of non-fat milk

Lunch

Preparation time: 10 minutes

Cooking time: 22 minutes

1 medium Roasted skinless chicken sandwich

½ cup Pasta salad

1 medium Pear

1 cup unsweetened Fruit juice

Pasta salad

Preparation time: 5 minutes

Cooking time: 3 minutes

Ingredients:

¼ cup Penne pasta noodles

¼ cup celery sliced thin, corn kernels and chopped fresh tarragon

1 teaspoon olive oil

A dash of black pepper and kosher salt

Directions:

Cook the penne pasta as stated by the directions on the package. Rinse beneath cold water, then drain. In a bowl, mix the pasta, corn kernels, celery and tarragon with the olive oil, salt and pepper.

Dinner

Salmon Pineapple Medley

Blue cheese and cherry salad

½ cup Brown rice

Glass of wine

Salmon Pineapple Medley

Preparation time: 2 minutes

Cooking time: 12 minutes

Ingredients:

1/4 cup chopped fresh pineapple

1/2 tablespoon red onion chopped fine

1/2 tablespoons chopped cilantro

1 teaspoon rice vinegar

A dash of ground red pepper and salt

Culinary spray

6 ounces salmon fillet, cut half inch thick

Directions:

Take pineapple, red onion, cilantro, vinegar and pepper inside a container. Set on the side. Heat a coated grill saucepan with culinary spray above medium-high temperature. Sprinkle salt over the fish and cook for four minutes on every side, or till it peels well once tested using a fork. Transfer atop a dinner plate and top with the salsa.

Snack

Baby carrots, 1/2 cup Homemade Peach ice cream, and 1 cup Water

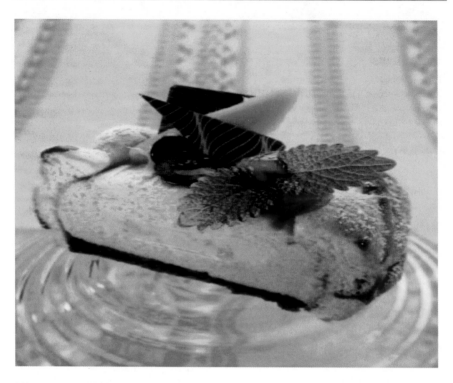

Homemade Peach Ice Cream

Preparation time: 2 hours

Ingredients:

1 cup evaporated fat-free milk

1/2 cup fat-free milk

1/3 cup calorie-free sweetener

1/4 cup egg substitute

1/8 teaspoon almond or vanilla extract

1/2 cup chopped fresh or frozen peaches

Directions:

Combine all the milk, sweetener, egg substitute and almond extract in a bowl. Beat with a blender at an average speed till smooth. Then, stir the peaches inside the bowl with the mixture. Pour the mixture in a freezer tin of an electric or hand-turned freezer. Freeze according to the instructions on the pack. Pack the freezer with extra rock salt and ice while letting it stand for at least an hour before serving.

Day 2 breakdown

Nutrition Facts	
	Amount
Calories	1793 Cal
Proteins	54 g
Fats	64 g
Saturated fats	12 g
Monounsaturated fats	38 g
Polyunsaturated fats	14 g
Cholesterol	109 mg
Carbohydrates	269 g
Fiber	38 g
Sodium	1098 mg

DAY 3

Breakfast

Preparation time: 3 minutes

Cooking time: 2 minutes

¾ cup Bran cereal with 1 medium Banana and 1 cup non-fat milk

1 medium Light Buttermilk Biscuit

1 cup Honeydew melon cubes

1 cup calcium fortified Orange juice

1 cup Coffee with 2 tablespoons non-fat milk

Light Buttermilk Biscuits

Preparation time: 40 minutes

Cooking time: 30 minutes

Ingredients:

1 cup all-purpose flour

2 teaspoons baking powder

1/4 teaspoon baking soda

1/4 teaspoon salt

1/2 cup buttermilk

1/4 cup canola oil

Directions:

Mix all dry parts together in a mixing container. In another bowl, blend together the oil and buttermilk, and then add it to the first mixture. Blend everything until just moistened. Knead the dough on a dusted surface by means of folding it in half, as well as pressing it a bit downward.

Next, make the dough to preferred thickness without overworking it. If you do, it will become hard. Cut the dough using a cutter and place them on a greased sheet. Then bake the cut biscuits at 450° for around nine minutes. Be watchful, so as not to over-bake them. When the top of the biscuits become a bit golden take the biscuits out of the oven. The undersides will be light brown. Serve piping hot with jelly or honey.

Lunch

Preparation time: 15 minutes

Cooking time: 1 hour

Baked chicken breast

½ cup Collard greens, cooked in a tablespoon of low-salt chicken broth

½ cup Black-eyed peas with 1 medium Corn on the cob coated with a teaspoon of soft margarine

1 cup cooked Rice topped with a teaspoon of soft margarine

1 cup of canned Fruit cocktail

1 cup unsweetened iced tea

Baked Chicken Breast

Ingredients:

3 ounces chicken breast

1/4 teaspoon Salt Substitute

2 teaspoon canola oil

Directions:

Remove the skin of the chicken and rub sodium substitute on the meat. Next place the chicken in a baking pan and brush the oil on top. Bake without cover for 45 minutes at 325° or till the juices turn clear.

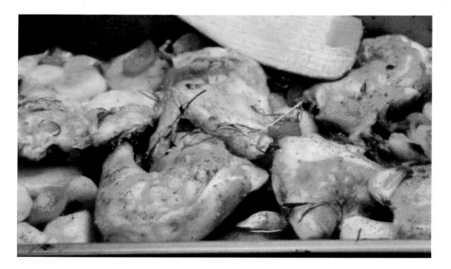

Dinner

Preparation time: 5 minutes

Cooking time: 20 minutes

Baked Breaded Catfish

1 medium Sweet potato with 2 teaspoons soft margarine

½ cup Spinach, cooked with 2 tablespoons low-salt vegetable soup

1 medium Corn muffin made using egg substitute, fat-free milk and a teaspoon of soft margarine

1 cup Watermelon cubes

1 cup unsweetened iced tea

Baked Breaded Catfish

Preparation time: 7 minutes

Cooking time: 12 minutes

Ingredients:

1 whisked egg, but use only ¼ of it

1/2 tablespoons lemon juice

1/8 cup all-purpose flour

1/4 teaspoon Cajun seasoning

1/8 teaspoon garlic powder

1/8 teaspoon salt

3 ounce catfish fillet

1/2 tablespoon canola oil

Directions:

In a shallow bowl, mix the lemon juice and egg. In a separate shallow container, combine the seasoning, flour, salt, and garlic powder. Dip the catfish in the egg mix, and then cover with the other mixture. In a baking pan, spread the oil and put the coated catfish on it. Bake at medium temperature for 12 minutes, or until the fish crumbles when tested using a fork.

Snack

1 medium Bagel with 1 tablespoon low-fat, salt-free Peanut butter, and 1 cup non-fat milk

Day 3 Nutrient breakdown:

Nutrition Facts	
	Amount
Calories	2504 Cal
Proteins	111 g
Fats	83 g
Saturated fats	17 g
Monounsaturated fats	38 g
Polyunsaturated fats	28 g
Cholesterol	158 mg
Carbohydrates	368 g
Fiber	52 g
Sodium	2147 mg

DAY 4

Breakfast

Preparation time: 7 minutes

Cooking time: 2 minutes

¾ cup Bran cereal with 1 medium Banana and 1 cup non-fat milk

1 medium low-salt Biscuit made using canola oil

1 tablespoon of jelly and a teaspoon of soft margarine

1/2 cup Honeydew melon cubes

1 cup Coffee with 2 tablespoons non-fat milk

Lunch

Preparation time: 7 minutes

Cooking time: 30 minutes

2 ounces Baked chicken breast

1 medium Corn on the cob coated with a teaspoon of soft margarine

½ cup Collard greens, cooked in a tablespoon of low-salt chicken broth

1 cup cooked Rice

1 cup of canned Fruit cocktail

1 cup unsweetened iced tea

Dinner

Preparation time: 12 minutes

Cooking time: 30 minutes

3 ounces Baked Breaded Catfish

1 medium Sweet potato with 2 teaspoons soft margarine

½ cup Spinach, cooked with 2 tablespoons low-salt vegetable soup

1 medium Corn muffin made using egg substitute, fat-free milk and a teaspoon of soft margarine

1 cup Watermelon cubes

1 cup unsweetened iced tea

Snack

Preparation time: 2 minutes

4 large Graham crackers and a tablespoon of low-fat

Salt-free Peanut butter and ½ cup non-fat milk

Day 4 Nutrient breakdown:

Nutrition Facts	
	Amount
Calories	1824 Cal
Proteins	111 g
Fats	61 g
Saturated fats	10 g
Monounsaturated fats	28 g
Polyunsaturated fats	16 g
Cholesterol	131 mg
Carbohydrates	272 g
Fiber	43 g
Sodium	1676 mg

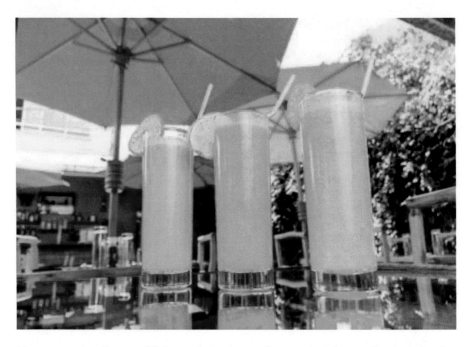

You may try these drink recipes to replace what is on the menu. It will alter the nutrient intake for the day.

Cranberry Grapefruit Sparklers

Preparation time: 15 minutes

Ingredients:

1 ¼ cups fresh grapefruit juice

1 ¾ cups chilled cranberry juice

1 1/4 cups chilled sparkling or soda water

1/2 lime, cut into small wedges

Directions:

Stir grapefruit and cranberry juices together in a large jug. Just before serving, mix in the water. Serve with ice and lime slices. This recipe serves four people. Each serving has: Calories – 88; Carbohydrate – 22 grams; and Sodium – 156 milligrams.

Orange Jewel

Preparation time: 5 minutes

Ingredients:

3 ounces frozen orange juice concentrate

1/4 cup sifted powdered sugar

1 cup skim milk

1/2 teaspoon vanilla

3 large ice cubes

Directions:

In a blender, mix the sugar, juice and milk, then cover, as well as blend till smooth. With the blender in motion, add the ice one after another. And put on the cover again to blend afterward add ice. Blend till frothy and then pour in three chilled goblets for serving. Each serving has 172 Calories.

5 grams protein, 37 grams carbohydrate, 2 mg cholesterol and 65 mg sodium

Minty Pineapple Lemonade

Preparation time: 5 minutes

Ingredients:

1 ½ cups pineapple juice

1 ½ juiced lemons

½ cup white sugar or Saccharin

¼ cup honey

3 slices lemon

1 liter bottle carbonated water

Fresh mint leaves

Directions:

To prepare the lemon-pineapple syrup:

In a big saucepan combine the honey, pineapple and lemon juices, and sugar. Raise heat over average. Boil for a minute and set aside to cool before refrigerating it overnight.

The next day, fill with ice three glasses, and place a lemon slice in every glass. Pour inside around two fluid ounces of the pineapple-lemon sweet liquid. Fill the glasses brimming with water and stir. Crush the fresh leaves of mint to garnish each glass before serving.

Nutrition Facts Per Serving		
Item	Sugar	Saccharin
Calories	313 Cal	123 Cal
Proteins	1 g	1 g
Carbohydrates	81 g	50 g
Fiber	1 g	1 g
Sodium	17 mg	17 mg

DAY 5

Breakfast

Preparation time: 5 minutes

Cooking time: 15 minutes

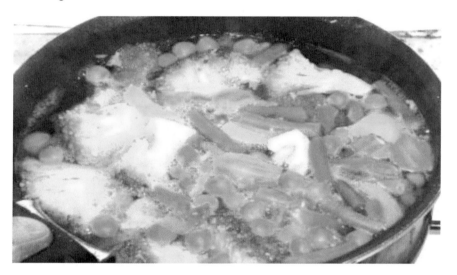

Bean Tortilla

1 medium Papaya

1 cup calcium fortified Orange Juice

1 cup Coffee with 2 tablespoons non-fat milk

Bean Tortilla

Preparation time: 5 minutes

Cooking time: 15 minutes

Ingredients:

1 teaspoon canola oil

¼ cup chopped onion

1/2 cup pinto or kidney beans, drained

1/4 cup chopped ripe tomatoes

1 medium Jalapeno pepper

2 flour or corn tortillas

Directions:

Heat the canola oil in the pan, besides cooking the onion for two minutes. Add the beans and heat for another three minutes. Mash in the onions using a fork towards making a coarse paste. Then, add the tomatoes and a tablespoon of water. Cover and boil 10 minutes over light heat. Keep stirring until it thickens and become pulpy. You must season with pepper while warming the tortillas in another dry pan. Fill, spin and enjoy the food!

Lunch

Preparation time: 10 minutes

Cooking time: 30 minutes

Stir-fried Beef

For Mexican rice we use 1 cup cooked rice

¼ cup chopped onion.

¼ cup chopped tomato

1 medium Jalapeno pepper along with ¼ cup diced carrots

2 tablespoons cilantro and a tablespoon of olive oil

1 medium Mango

1 cup Blended fruit drink using 1 cup non-fat milk, ¼ cup diced mango, ¼ cup sliced Banana, and ¼ cup of water

Ingredients:

3 ounces Sirloin steak

1 teaspoon minced Garlic

¼ cup chopped Onion

¼ cup chopped Tomatoes

1/4 cup diced Potato

1/4 cup Salsa

2 teaspoons Olive oil

Directions:

Heat a wok or heavy-based cooking pan till warm and add the olive oil. Next, stir-fry the slices of beef with the garlic, onion, tomato and potato until cooked. Serve with salsa on the side.

Dinner

Chicken fajita

Avocado salad using 1 cup Romaine lettuce

1 small sliced dark skinned Avocado

¼ cup sliced Tomato; 2 tablespoons chopped Onion; and 1 ½ tablespoons low-fat Sour cream

¾ cup Rice pudding with raisins

1 cup Water

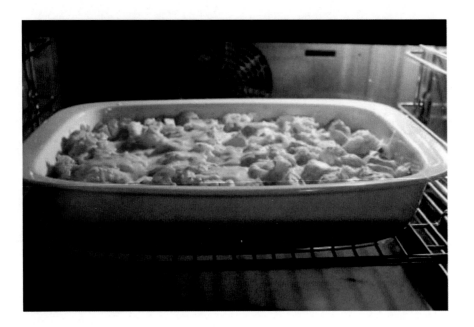

Preparation time: 10 minutes

Cooking time: 12 minutes

Ingredients:

3 ounces baked chicken breast

2 tablespoons chopped onion

2 teaspoons canola oil

¼ cup chopped Green pepper

1 teaspoon minced Garlic

2 tablespoons Salsa

2 medium corn tortillas

Directions:

You have already marinated and baked the chicken. It is time to stir-fry the onions, pepper and garlic in canola oil for a minute over high heat. Put in the chicken and use an iron spatula to collect the fried bits. Spread the peppers and onions in a smooth layer inside the cooking pan. Allow them to cook for two minutes. Make sure to cut the chicken into narrow pieces. Serve immediately with the warm tortillas and salsa.

Snack

1 cup unsweetened non-fat Plain yogurt with ½ cup peaches and 1 cup water.

Day 5 Nutrient Breakdown:

Nutrition Facts Per Serving	Amount
Calories	2613 Cal
Proteins	111 g
Fats	81 g
Saturated fats	15 g
Monounsaturated fats	47 g
Polyunsaturated fats	19 g
Cholesterol	157 mg
Carbohydrates	379 g
Fiber	50 g
Sodium	2090 mg

DAY 6

Breakfast

Preparation time: 5 minutes

Cooking time: 20 minutes

1 Bean Tortilla

1 medium Papaya

1 cup calcium fortified Orange Juice

1 cup Coffee with 2 tablespoons non-fat milk

Lunch

Preparation time: 5 minutes

Cooking time: 40 minutes

2 ounces Stir-fried Beef

Mexican rice using 1/2 cup cooked rice

2 tablespoons chopped onion

2 tablespoons chopped tomato

1 medium Jalapeno pepper

2 tablespoons diced carrots, 1 tablespoons cilantro, and 2 tablespoons of olive oil

1 medium Mango

1 cup Blended fruit drink using 1 cup non-fat milk, ¼ cup diced mango, 1/4 cup sliced Banana, and 1/4 cup of water

Dinner

Preparation time: 12 minutes

Cooking time: 13 minutes

2 ounces Chicken fajita with only one corn tortilla

Avocado salad using 1 cup Romaine lettuce

1/2 small sliced dark skinned Avocado

¼ cup sliced Tomato; 2 tablespoons chopped Onion; and 1 ½ tablespoons low-fat Sour cream

1/2 cup Rice pudding with raisins

1 cup Water

Snack

1 cup unsweetened non-fat Plain yogurt mixed with ½ cup Peaches, and a cup of Water

Day 6 Nutrient breakdown:

Nutrition Facts Per Serving	
	Amount
Calories	1821 Cal
Proteins	77 g
Fats	53 g
Saturated fats	9 g
Monounsaturated fats	36 g
Polyunsaturated fats	8 g
Cholesterol	109 mg
Carbohydrates	278 g
Fiber	32 g
Sodium	1739 mg

You have stuck with the diet with great difficulty, I suppose. Now it is time to reward yourself. Here is a low-fat dessert recipe you may incorporate in your daily food.

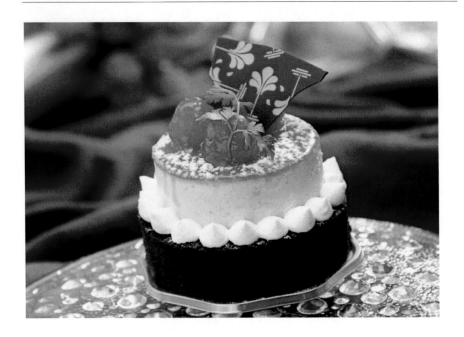

Elegant Chocó Raspberry Torte

Preparation time: 30 minutes

Cooking time: 40 minutes

Ingredients:

3 tablespoons light corn oil spread

½ cup sugar

½ cup skim milk

½ tablespoon white vinegar

¼ teaspoon vanilla extract

¾ cups all-purpose flour

¼ cup Cocoa

½ teaspoon baking soda

1/8 cup red raspberry jam

Directions:

Heat the oven at 350°F. Spray a jelly roll cooking pan using vegetable spray. In a medium pan over a little heat, melt corn oil spread and mix in the sugar. Next, remove it from the heat and blend in the vanilla, vinegar and milk. In a small bowl, beat together the baking soda, cocoa, and flour. Then add it to the sugar mix.

Stir with a whisk till well mixed before pouring it into the prepared cooking pan. Bake for 17 minutes, or till a wooden stick inserted at the center appears clean when taken out. Cool for 10 minutes before removing from the pan to the wire stand. Cool and cut the cake into four parts.

Place a piece atop a serving platter and spread a tablespoon of jam above. Place 3/4 cup of Raspberry cream on top of the jam. Repeat the procedure using the remaining layers of cake, jam and the Raspberry cream. Stop with a plain top layer. Spread the remaining jam on top and spoon the rest of the Raspberry cream above the jam. Refrigerate the torte. It is ready to serve seven people.

Thaw a package of 10 ounces iced up raspberries. This is to make the raspberry cream. Place the red raspberries in a mixer and blend until it is completely juiced. Strain using a sieve while discarding the pips. In a small mixing bowl, mix around 1.3 ounces of whipped coating mixture without water. Add half a cup of chilled skim milk, with vanilla and three drops of red food coloring, if preferred.

Nutrition Facts Per Serving	
	Amount
Calories	172 Cal
Proteins	3 g
Fats	3 g
Calcium	40 mg
Carbohydrates	34 g
Fiber	32 g
Sodium	110 mg

DAY 7

Breakfast

Preparation time: 10 minutes

Cooking time: 2 minutes

Scrambled egg white - use half a cup of liquid egg substitute and cook with fat-free cooking spray

1 whole English muffin topped with two teaspoons of soft margarine and a tablespoon of jam

1 cup strawberries

1 cup calcium fortified orange juice

1 cup coffee with two tablespoons of fat-free milk

Lunch

Preparation time: 2 minutes

Cooking time: 30 minutes

Stir-fried Tofu Veggies

½ cup cooked rice

1 medium orange

1 cup green tea

Stir-fried Tofu Veggies

Preparation time: 15 minutes

Cooking time: 20 minutes

Ingredients:

3 ounces extra firm tofu

½ cup roughly cut mushrooms

½ cup onions

½ cup diced carrots

½ cup Swiss chard

2 tablespoons minced garlic

1tablespoon peanut oil

2 ½ teaspoons low-salt soy sauce

Directions:

Preheat oven to 400. Dry the tofu. Drain, detach from the pack, and put between two towels doubled over it. Then, you can position a bowl atop it with a book while letting it drip for around a quarter of an hour. Change the towels when they become too damp. Wait for it to dry. Chop into 1 inch cubes.

Next, arrange the tofu over a greased baking piece to avert sticking. Bake it for 30 minutes, overturning once midway through to ensure even heating. This would dry off the tofu, besides help in giving an extra meaty feel. If you wish a rougher texture, heat it for 35 minutes. Or else, 20 minutes should do.

Once golden in color and firm, remove from the oven. Set aside to cool for close to an hour. Take a skillet and heat above medium-high temperature. Add the oil and veggies tossing and stirring often for six minutes. When the veggies have softened a little, add the soy sauce. Keep stirring.

When it starts to thicken, add the tofu. Cover it with the sauce and simmer for four minutes. Turn off the heat and serve on top of rice or have it as it is. It is best when consumed fresh, but will hold in the fridge for a few days.

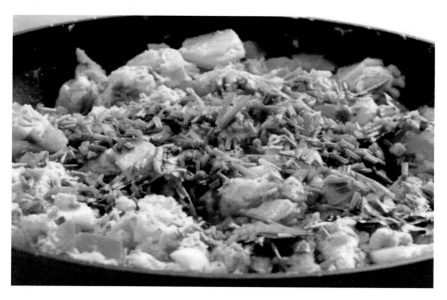

Dinner

Preparation time: 5 minutes

Cooking time: 1 hour

Beef stir-fry using three ounces beef tenderloin

¼ cup cooked soybeans

Half cup large pieces of broccoli, a tablespoon of peanut oil, and two teaspoons of low-salt soy sauce

Half cup cooked rice

1 cup watermelon cubes

1 Almond cookie

1 cup non-fat milk

Snack

½ cup Chinese noodles with a teaspoon of peanut oil, and a cup of green tea

Day 7 Nutrient Breakdown

Nutrition Facts Per Serving	
	Amount
Calories	1963 Cal
Proteins	88 g
Fats	57 g
Saturated fats	13 g
Monounsaturated fats	22 g
Polyunsaturated fats	22 g
Cholesterol	73 mg
Carbohydrates	256 g
Fiber	29 g
Sodium	1789 mg

ONE LAST THING…

If you enjoyed this book or found it useful I'd be very grateful if you left a review. Your support makes all the difference and I read all of your reviews personally so I can get feedback to make this book (and my future books) even better.

If you would like to sign up to read my latest work and get your hands on some FREE eBooks then head over to TimothyPyke.com

Made in the USA
Las Vegas, NV
04 January 2023

64861904R00045